The Super Easy Lean & Green Cookbook

Easy And Delicious Lean & green Recipes For Beginners

Jesse Cohen

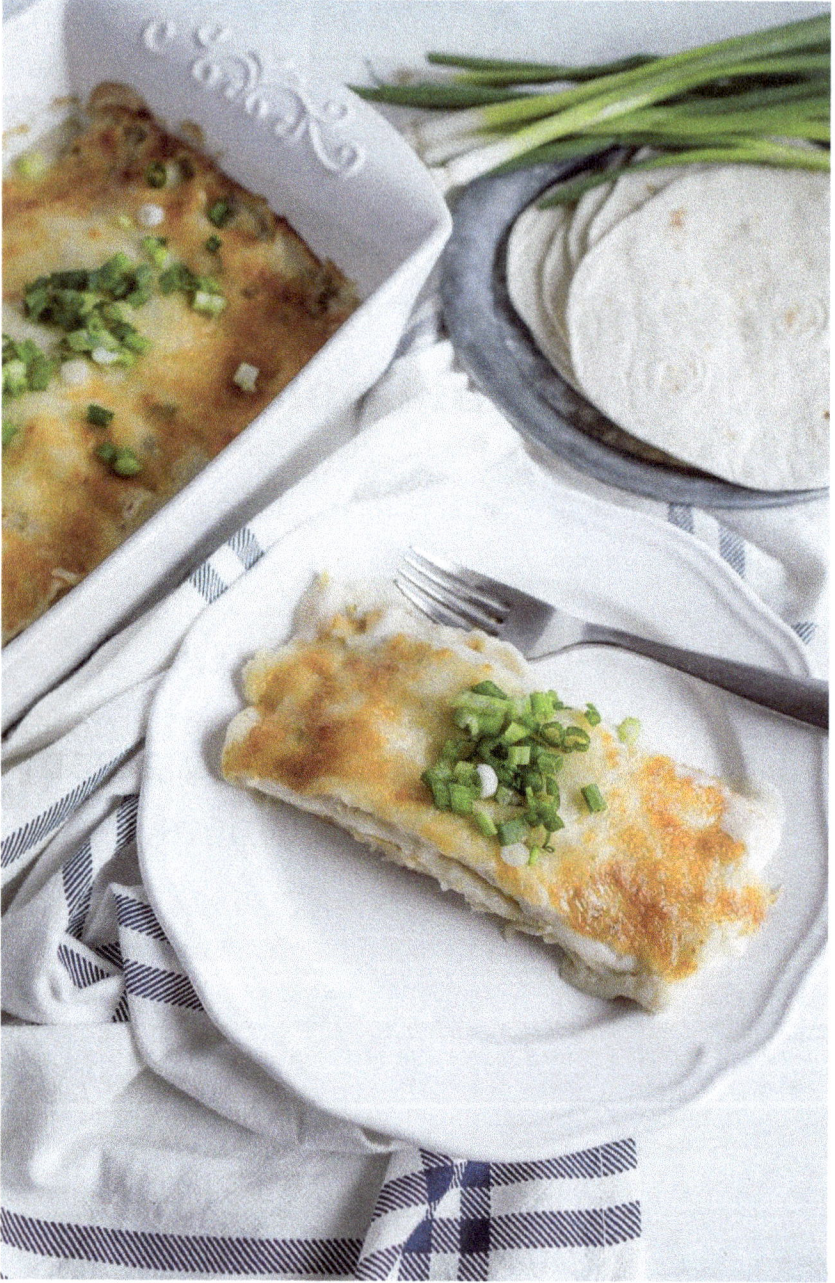

Table of contents

5

6

Cheesy Egg Veggie Omelet

Preparation Time: 5 minutes

Cooking Time: 6 minutes

Servings: 2

Ingredients:

- 3 eggs
- 1/2 cup of cheddar cheese; grated
- 2 garlic cloves; minced
- 1 tbsp. of parsley; chopped
- Sea salt and pepper to taste
- 2 tbsp. of mozzarella cheese; grated
- 1 tbsp. of olive oil

Directions:

1. Whisk the eggs in a bowl. Add some salt and pepper.
2. Heat the olive oil in a pan.
3. Add the garlic and toss for 1 minute.
4. Add the egg mixture and cook for 1 minute.
5. Add the cheddar, parsley, and parmesan cheese.

6. Fold the egg in half and cook for an additional minute.

7. Serve hot.

Nutrition:

- Protein: 21.7 g
- Carbohydrates: 9.1 g
- Dietary Fiber: 1.6 g
- Sugars: 4.8 g
- Fat: 29.8 g

Chicken & Pepperoni Pizza

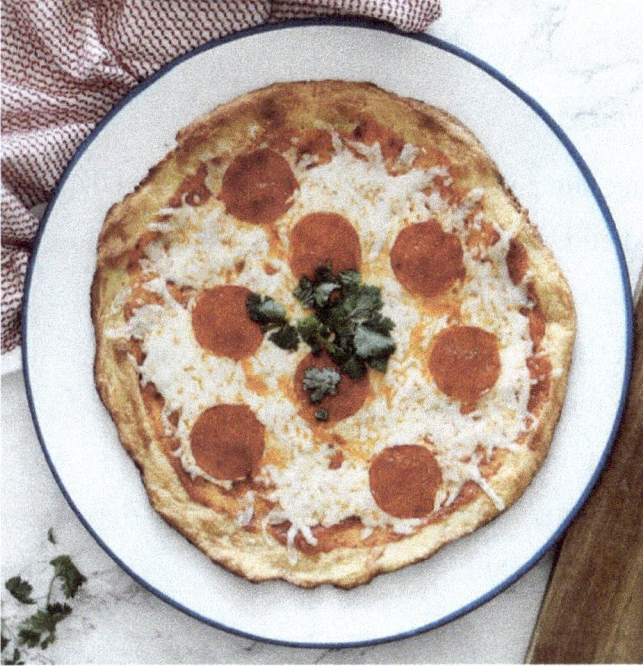

Preparation Time: 5 minutes

Cooking Time: 15 minutes

Servings: 6

Ingredients:

- 2 cups of cooked chicken; cubed

- 20 slices of pepperoni

- 1 cup of sugar-free pizza sauce

- 1 cup of mozzarella cheese; shredded
- ¼ cup of parmesan cheese; grated

Directions:

1. Place the chicken at the bottom of a four-cup baking dish and add the pepperoni and pizza sauce on top. Mix well so as to coat the meat with the sauce completely.
2. Add the parmesan and mozzarella on top of the chicken, then place the baking dish into your fryer.
3. Cook for 15 minutes at 375°F.
4. When everything is bubbling and melted, remove from the fryer. Serve hot.

Nutrition:

- Calories: 239
- Fat: 12 g
- Carbs: 8 g
- Protein: 11 g

Chicken Burgers

Preparation Time: 15 minutes

Cooking Time: 15 minutes

Servings: 4

Ingredients:

- 8 oz. of ground chicken
- 1 cup of fresh spinach; blended
- 1 teaspoon of minced onion
- ½ teaspoon of salt
- 1 red bell pepper; grinded
- 1 egg; beaten
- 1 teaspoon of ground black pepper
- 4 tablespoons of Panko breadcrumbs

Directions:

1. In a bowl, mix together the ground chicken, blended spinach, minced garlic, salt, grinded bell pepper, egg, and ground black pepper.

2. When the chicken mixture is smooth, make 4 burgers from it and coat them in Panko breadcrumbs.
3. Place the burgers in the non-sticky baking dish or line the baking tray with baking paper.
4. Bake the burgers for 15 minutes at 365° F.
5. Flip the chicken burgers on another side after 7 minutes of cooking.

Nutrition:

- Calories: 177
- Fat: 5.2 g
- Fiber: 1.8 g
- Carbs: 10.4 g
- Protein: 13.2 g

Chicken Saute

Preparation Time: 10 minutes

Cooking Time: 25 minutes

Servings: 2

Ingredients:

- 4 oz. of chicken fillet
- 4 tomatoes; peeled
- 1 bell pepper, chopped
- 1 teaspoon of olive oil
- 1 cup of water
- 1 teaspoon of salt
- 1 chili pepper; chopped
- ½ teaspoon of saffron

Directions:

1. Pour water in the pan and bring it to a boil.
2. Meanwhile, chop the chicken fillet.
3. Add the chicken fillet in the boiling water and cook it for 10 minutes or until the chicken is soft.

4. After this, put the chopped bell pepper and chili pepper in the skillet.
5. Add olive oil and roast the vegetables for 3 minutes.
6. Add chopped tomatoes and blend up well.
7. Cook the vegetables for 2 more minutes.
8. Then add salt and a ¾ cup of water from boiling chicken.
9. Add chopped chicken fillet and blend up.
10. Cook the sauté for 10 minutes over the medium heat.

Nutrition:

- Calories: 192
- Fat: 7.2 g
- Fiber: 3.8 g
- Carbs: 14.4 g
- Protein: 19.2 g

Italian Chicken Thighs

Preparation Time: 10 minutes

Cooking Time: 20 minutes

Servings: 4

Ingredients:

- 4 skin-on bone-in chicken thighs
- 2 tbsps. of unsalted butter; melted
- 3 tsps. of Italian herbs
- ½ tsp. of garlic powder
- ¼ tsp. of onion powder

Directions:

1. Using a brush, coat the chicken thighs with the melted butter. Mix the herbs with the garlic powder and onion powder, then massage into the chicken thighs. Place the thighs in the fryer.
2. Cook at 380°F for 20 minutes, turning the chicken halfway through to cook on the other side.

3. When the thighs have attained a golden color, test the temperature with a thermometer. Once it reaches 165°F, remove from the fryer and serve.

Nutrition:

- Calories: 265
- Fat: 21 g
- Carbs: 22 g
- Protein: 32 g

Chicken Loaf

Preparation Time: 10 minutes

Cooking Time: 40 minutes

Servings: 4

Ingredients:

- 2 cups of ground chicken
- 1 egg, beaten
- 1 tablespoon of fresh dill; chopped
- 1 garlic clove; chopped
- ½ teaspoon of salt
- 1 teaspoon of chili flakes
- 1 onion; minced

Directions:

1. In a bowl, mix together all the ingredients and blend up until you get smooth mass.
2. Then line the loaf dish with baking paper and put the bottom chicken mixture inside.
3. Flatten the surface well.

4. Bake the chicken loaf for 40 minutes at 355° F.

5. Then chill the chicken loaf to the room temperature and take away from the loaf dish.

6. Slice it.

Nutrition:

- Calories: 167
- Fat: 6.2 g
- Fiber: 0.8 g
- Carbs: 3.4 g
- Protein: 32.2 g

Creamy Chicken Pate

Preparation Time: 2 hours

Cooking Time: 20 minutes

Servings: 6

Ingredients:

- 8 oz. of chicken liver
- 3 tablespoon of butter
- 1 white onion; chopped
- 1 bay leaf
- 1 teaspoon of salt
- ½ teaspoon of ground black pepper
- ½ cup of water

Directions:

1. Place the liver in the saucepan.
2. Add onion, bay leaf, salt, ground black pepper, and water.
3. Mix up the mixture and shut the lid.
4. Cook the liver mixture for 20 minutes over medium heat.
5. Then transfer it in the blender and blend until smooth.

6. Add butter and blend up until it is melted.

7. Pour the pate mixture in the pate ramekin and refrigerate for 2 hours.

Nutrition:

- Calories: 122
- Fat: 8.2 g
- Fiber: 0.8 g
- Carbs: 2.4 g
- Protein: 9.2 g

Arugula Fig Chicken

Preparation Time: 15 minutes

Cooking Time: 30 minutes

Servings: 4

Ingredients:

- 2 teaspoons of cornstarch

- 2 cloves of garlic; crushed

- ¾ cup of Mission figs; chopped

- ¼ cup of black or green olives; chopped

- 1 bag of baby arugula

- ½ cup of chicken broth

- 8 skinless chicken thighs

- 2 teaspoons of olive oil

- 2 teaspoons of brown sugar

- ½ cup of red wine vinegar

- Ground black pepper and salt; to taste

Directions:

1. Over medium stove flame, heat the oil in a skillet or saucepan (preferably of medium size).
2. Add the chicken, sprinkle with some salt and cook until evenly brown. Set it aside.
3. Add and sauté the garlic.
4. In a bowl, mix the vinegar, broth, cornstarch, and sugar. Add the mixture into the pan and simmer until the sauce thickens.
5. Add the figs and olives; simmer for a couple of minutes. Serve warm with chopped arugula on top.

Nutrition:

- Calories: 364
- Fat: 14 g
- Carbohydrates: 29 g
- Fiber: 5 g
- Protein: 31 g

Parmesan Chicken Gratin

Preparation Time: 10 minutes

Cooking Time: 30 minutes

Servings: 4

Ingredients:

- 2 chicken thighs; skinless, boneless
- 1 teaspoon of paprika
- 1 tablespoon of lemon juice
- ½ teaspoon of chili flakes
- ¼ teaspoon of garlic powder
- 3 oz. of Parmesan; grated
- 1/3 cup of milk
- 1 onion; sliced
- 2 oz. of pineapple; sliced

Directions:

1. Chop the chicken thighs roughly and sprinkle them with paprika, lemon juice, chili flakes, garlic powder, and blend up well.

23

2. Arrange the chopped chicken thighs in the baking dish in one layer.

3. Then place sliced onion over the chicken.

4. Add the layer of sliced pineapple.

5. Mix together the milk and Parmesan and pour the liquid over the pineapple.

6. Cover the surface of the baking dish with foil and bake gratin for 30 minutes at 355° F.

Nutrition:

- Calories: 100
- Fat: 5.2
- Fiber: 1 g
- Carbs: 6.7 g
- Protein: 8.1 g

Grilled Marinated Chicken

Preparation Time: 35 minutes

Cooking Time: 20 minutes

Servings: 6

Ingredients:

- 2 pound of chicken breast; skinless, boneless
- 2 tablespoons of lemon juice
- 1 teaspoon of sage
- ½ teaspoon of ground nutmeg
- ½ teaspoon of dried oregano
- 1 teaspoon of paprika
- 1 teaspoon of onion powder
- 2 tablespoons of olive oil
- 1 teaspoon of chili flakes
- 1 teaspoon of salt
- 1 teaspoon of apple cider vinegar

Directions:

1. Preparing the marinade: whisk together apple vinegar, salt, chili flakes, olive oil, onion powder, paprika, dried oregano, ground nutmeg, sage, and lemon juice.
2. Then rub the chicken with marinade carefully and leave for 25 minutes to marinate.
3. Meanwhile, preheat grill to 385° F.
4. Place the marinated chicken breast in the grill and cook it for 10 minutes from all sides.
5. Cut the cooked chicken on the servings.

Nutrition:

- Calories: 218
- Fat: 8.2 g
- Fiber: 0.8 g
- Carbs: 0.4 g
- Protein: 32.2 g

Chicken Fillets with Artichoke Hearts

Preparation Time: 10 minutes

Cooking Time: 30 minutes

Servings: 3

Ingredients:

- 1 can of artichoke hearts; chopped

- 12 oz. of chicken fillets (3 oz. each fillet)

- 1 teaspoon of avocado oil

- ½ teaspoon of ground thyme

- ½ teaspoon of white pepper

- 1/3 cup of water

- 1/3 cup of shallot; roughly chopped

- 1 lemon; sliced

Directions:

1. Mix together the chicken fillets, artichoke hearts, avocado oil, ground thyme, white pepper, and shallot.

2. Line the baking tray with baking paper and place the chicken fillet mixture in it.

3. Then add sliced lemon and water.

4. Bake the meal for 30 minutes at 375° F. Stir the ingredients while cooking to avoid burning.

Nutrition:

- Calories: 267
- Fat: 8.2 g
- Fiber: 3.8 g
- Carbs: 10.4 g
- Protein: 35.2 g

Chicken Meatballs with Carrot

Preparation Time: 10 minutes

Cooking Time: 10 minutes

Servings: 8

Ingredients:

- 1/3 cup of carrot; grated
- 1 onion; diced
- 2 cups of ground chicken
- 1 tablespoon of semolina
- 1 egg; beaten
- ½ teaspoon of salt
- 1 teaspoon of dried oregano
- 1 teaspoon of dried cilantro
- 1 teaspoon of chili flakes
- 1 tablespoon of coconut oil

Directions:

In a bowl, mix together the grated carrot, diced onion, ground chicken, semolina, egg, salt, dried oregano, cilantro, and chili flakes.

Make the meatballs with the help of a scooper.

Heat up the coconut oil in the skillet.

When it starts to shimmer, put meatballs in it.

Cook the meatballs for 5 minutes from all sides over the medium-low heat.

Nutrition:

- Calories: 107
- Fat: 4.2 g
- Fiber: 0.8 g
- Carbs: 2.4 g
- Protein: 11.2 g

Duck Patties

Preparation Time: 15 minutes

Cooking Time: 10 minutes

Servings: 8

Ingredients:

- 1-pound of duck breast; skinless, boneless
- 1 teaspoon of semolina
- ½ teaspoon of cayenne pepper
- 2 eggs; beaten
- 1 teaspoon of salt
- 1 tablespoon of fresh cilantro; chopped
- 1 tablespoon of olive oil

Directions:

1. Chop the duck breast into small pieces (grind it) and mix alongside semolina, cayenne pepper, salt, and cilantro. Mix well.
2. Then add the eggs and stir gently.
3. Pour olive oil in the skillet and heat it up.

4. Place the duck mixture in the oil with the help of the spoon to make the form of small patties.

5. Fry the patties for 3 minutes from all sides over the medium heat.

6. Then close the lid and cook patties for 4 minutes more over the low heat.

Nutrition:

- Calories 106
- Fat: 5.2 g
- Fiber: 0.8 g
- Carbs: 0.4 g
- Protein: 13.2 g

Curry Chicken Drumsticks

Preparation Time: 10 minutes

Cooking Time: 30 minutes

Servings: 4

Ingredients:

- 4 chicken drumsticks
- 1 apple; grated
- 1 tablespoon of curry paste
- 4 tablespoons of milk
- 1 teaspoon of coconut oil
- 1 teaspoon of chili flakes
- ½ teaspoon of minced ginger

Directions:

1. Mix up together grated apple, curry paste, milk, chili flakes, and minced garlic.
2. Put coconut oil in the skillet and melt it.
3. Add apple mixture and stir well.
4. Then add chicken drumsticks and blend up well.

5. Roast the chicken for two minutes from all sides.

6. Then preheat oven to 360° F.

7. Place the skillet with chicken drumsticks in the oven and bake for 25 minutes.

Nutrition:

- Calories: 152
- Fat: 7.2 g
- Fiber: 1.8 g
- Carbs: 9.4 g
- Protein: 13.2 g

Chicken Enchiladas

Preparation Time: 20 minutes

Cooking Time: 15 minutes

Servings: 5

Ingredients:

- 5 corn tortillas

- 10 oz. of chicken breast; boiled, shredded

- 1 teaspoon of chipotle pepper

- 3 tablespoons of green salsa

- ½ teaspoon of minced garlic

- ½ cup of cream

- ¼ cup of chicken stock

- 1 cup of Mozzarella; shredded

- 1 teaspoon of butte; softened

Directions:

1. Mix together the shredded chicken breast, chipotle pepper, green salsa, and minced garlic.

2. Then put the shredded chicken mixture in the center of each corn tortilla and roll them.
3. Spread softened butter on the inside of the baking dish and arrange the rolled corn tortillas.
4. Then pour chicken broth and cream over the tortillas.
5. Top them with shredded Mozzarella.
6. Bake the enchiladas for 15 minutes at 365° F.

Nutrition:

- Calories: 152
- Fat: 5.2 g
- Fiber: 1.8 g
- Carbs: 12.4 g
- Protein: 15.2 g

Chicken Fajitas

Preparation Time: 15 minutes

Cooking Time: 15 minutes

Servings: 2

Ingredients:

- 1 bell pepper

- ½ red onion; peeled

- 5 oz. of chicken fillets

- 1 garlic clove; sliced

- 1 tablespoon of olive oil

- 1 teaspoon of balsamic vinegar

- 1 teaspoon of chili pepper

- ½ teaspoon of salt

- 1 teaspoon of lemon juice

- 2 flour tortillas

Directions:

1. Cut the bell pepper and chicken fillet on the wedges.

2. Then slice the onion.

3. Pour olive oil in the skillet and heat it up.

4. Add chicken wedges and sprinkle them with chili pepper and salt.

5. Roast the chicken for 4 minutes. Stir it from time to time.

6. After this, add juice and balsamic vinegar. Mix well.

7. Add bell pepper, onion, and clove.

8. Roast fajitas for 10 minutes over the medium-high heat. Stir it from time to time.

9. Put the cooked fajitas on the tortillas and transfer in the serving plates.

Nutrition:

- Calories: 346
- Fat: 14.2 g
- Fiber: 2.8 g
- Carbs: 23.4 g
- Protein: 25.2 g

Cashew Thai Beef Stir-Fry

Preparation Time: 5 minutes

Cooking Time: 30 minutes

Servings: 4

Ingredients:

- 2 cloves of garlic; crushed

- 5 tablespoons of lime juice

- 1 tablespoon of rice wine vinegar

- ½ teaspoon of cayenne pepper

- 2 teaspoons of soy sauce

- 2 sirloin steaks; either New York strip or top sirloin, about 1 pound each, cut into large strips

- 2 tablespoons of sesame oil

- 2 onions; diced

- 2 organic bell peppers; sliced into thin strips

- 1 cup of broccoli; chopped into florets

- ½ cup of cashews

- 2 tablespoons of grapeseed oil

Directions:

1. Mix garlic, lime juice, rice vinegar, cayenne pepper, and soy sauce. Set aside.
2. Brush the meat with the sesame oil. On high heat, add the grapeseed oil in the wok and when it is hot, fry the meat in two batches until it is browned and cooked. Remove from the wok and put aside.
3. Sauté onions until they are soft. Add peppers and broccoli and cook for 4 minutes. Add cashews and cook for 2 minutes.
4. Put the meat back in and cook until it is warm. Serve with rice if you desire.

Nutrition:

- Calories: 253
- Fat: 27 g
- Carbs: 36 g
- Protein: 12 g

Pineapple-BBQ Pork

Preparation Time: 10 minutes

Cooking Time: 6 minutes

Servings: 4

Ingredients:

- 4 bone-in pork loin chops
- One 8-ounce can of undrained crushed pineapple
- 1 cup of honey BBQ sauce
- 2 tablespoons of chili sauce
- 1 tablespoon of olive oil

Directions:

1. Mix can of pineapple, BBQ sauce, and condiment.
2. Turn your PPCXL to "chicken/meat" and heat.
3. When hot, add olive oil.
4. When the oil is sizzling, roast pork chops on each side, 3-4 minutes per side.
5. When brown, pour sauce over the pork and seal the lid.
6. Adjust time to six minutes.

7. When the time is up, hit "cancel" and wait 5 minutes before quick-releasing.

8. Pork should be cooked to 145° F.

9. Serve with sauce.

Nutrition:

- Total calories: 370
- Protein: 28 g
- Carbs: 37 g
- Fat: 13 g
- Fiber: 0

Brown Sugar Italian Pork

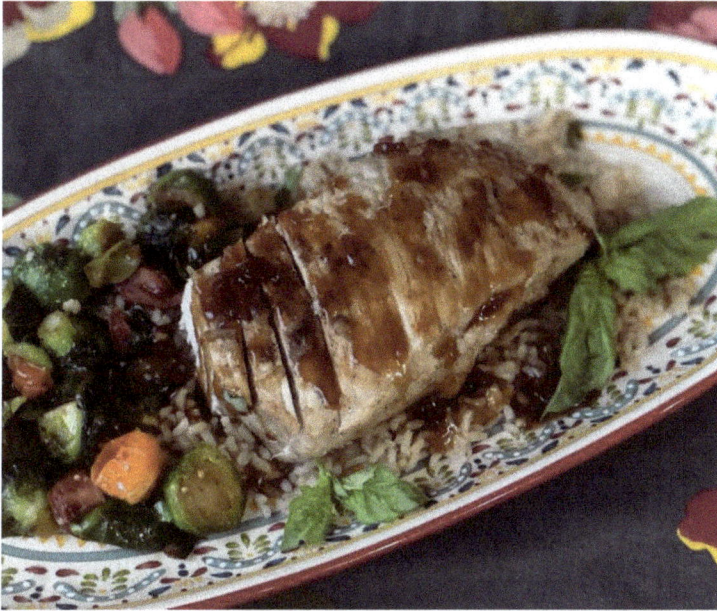

Preparation Time: 15 minutes

Cooking Time: 6 minutes

Servings: 6

Ingredients:

- 6 boneless pork chops

- ¾ cup of white wine

- ½ cup of brown sugar

- 3 tablespoons of Italian seasoning
- 1 tablespoon of olive oil

Directions:

1. Heat olive oil in your cooker with the lid off, on the "chicken/meat" setting.
2. While that heats up, season pork generously with Italian seasoning and brown sugar.
3. Add pork to cooker and roast on each side till golden.
4. Pour in wine and seal the lid.
5. Adjust cook time to 6 minutes.
6. When time is up, hit "cancel" and quick-release.
7. Make sure pork has reached 145° F.
8. Rest for 5 minutes before serving!

Nutrition:

- Total calories: 315
- Protein: 23 g
- Carbs: 27 g
- Fat: 13 g
- Fiber: 0

Pork with Cranberry-Honey Gravy

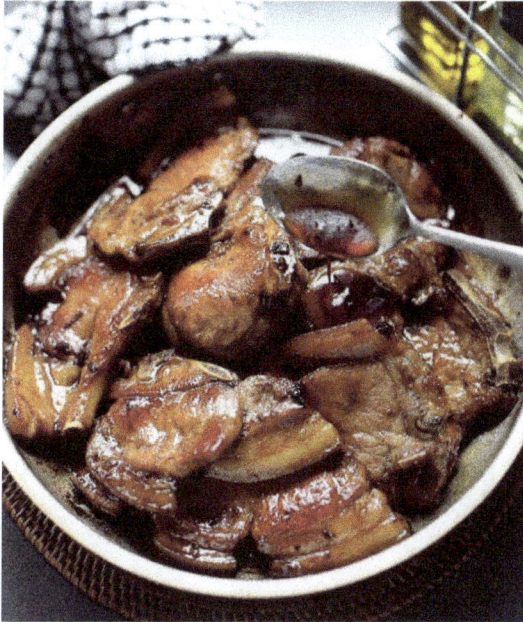

Preparation Time: 10 minutes

Cooking Time: 72 minutes

Servings: 4

Ingredients:

- 2 ½ pounds of bone-in pork shoulder

- 1 15-ounce can of whole-berry cranberry sauce

- ¼ cup of minced onion

- ¼ cup of honey
- Salt to taste

Directions:

1. Add all the ingredients into your pressure cooker and seal the lid.
2. Hit "chicken/meat" and adjust time to 1 hour, 12 minutes.
3. When the time is up, hit "cancel" and wait 10 minutes for a natural pressure release.
4. Remove the shoulder and de-bone.
5. Serve pork with gravy!

Nutrition:

- Total calories: 707
- Protein: 43 g
- Carbs: 61 g
- Fat: 30 g
- Fiber: 0

Lightened-Up Bangers & Mash

Preparation Time: 3 minutes

Cooking Time: 20 minutes

Servings: 6

Ingredients:

- 6 (4-ounce) pork sausages (raw)
- 3 pounds of peeled and diced butternut squash
- 1 cup of chicken broth
- 1 chopped onion
- 1 tablespoon of Dijon mustard

Directions:

1. To prep, poke the sausages a couple of times.
2. Put squash in the pot and pour in the cup of chicken broth.
3. Stir in the Dijon.
4. Add steamer basket and pile in sausages with onion on top.
5. Seal the lid.
6. Hit "chicken/meat" and adjust time to 20 minutes.
7. When the time is up, hit "cancel" and quick-release.

8. Sausage should be cooked to 145° F, while the squash is soft.

9. Serve!

Nutrition:

- Total calories: 506
- Protein: 19 g
- Carbs: 29 g
- Fat: 36 g
- Fiber: 5 g

Mexican-Braised Pork with Sweet Potatoes

Preparation Time: 10 minutes

Cooking Time: 25 minutes

Servings: 4

Ingredients:

- 3 pounds of pork loin
- 2 peeled and diced sweet potatoes
- 1 cup of tomato salsa
- ½ cup of chicken stock
- 1/3 cup of Mexican spice blend

Directions:

1. Season the pork all over with the spice blend.
2. Turn your cooker to "chicken/meat" and heat.
3. When hot, roast the pork on each side. If the meat sticks, pour in a little chicken broth.
4. When the pork is golden, pour in the salsa.
5. Tumble sweet potatoes on one side of the pot and seal the lid.

6. Adjust time to 25 minutes.

7. When the timer beeps, hit "cancel" and wait 10 minutes before quick-releasing.

8. The pork should be cooked to 145° F, and the potatoes should be soft.

9. Remove the pork and rest 8-10 minutes before serving.

Nutrition:

- Total calories: 513
- Protein: 73 g
- Carbs: 17 g
- Fat: 14 g
- Fiber: 1 g

Apricot-Glazed Pork Chops

Preparation Time: 15 minutes

Cooking Time: 6 minutes

Servings: 6

Ingredients:

- 6 boneless pork chops
- ½ cup of apricot
- 1 tablespoon of balsamic vinegar
- 2 teaspoons of olive oil
- Black pepper to taste

Directions:

1. Add oil to your cooker and heat on "chicken/meat," leaving the lid off.
2. Sprinkle black pepper on the pork chops.
3. Roast chops in the cooker on each side till golden.
4. Mix balsamic and apricot preserving together.
5. Pour over the pork and seal the cooker lid.
6. Adjust cook time to 6 minutes.
7. When the time is up, hit "cancel" and quick-release.

8. Test temperature of pork—it should be 145° F.

9. Allow to rest for 5 minutes before serving!

Nutrition:

- Total calories: 296
- Protein: 20 g
- Carbs: 18 g
- Fat: 16 g
- Fiber: 0

Simple Beef Stir-fry

Cooking Time: 30 minutes

Servings: 4

Ingredients:

- 2 cups of vegetable stock

- 2 tablespoons of soy sauce

- 4 garlic cloves; chopped

- 2 teaspoons of chili powder

- 1 pound of top sirloin beef; thinly sliced

- 3 cups of broccoli; chopped into florets

- 1 cup of cremini mushrooms; sliced

- 1 cup of sugar snaps peas

- 4 green onions; sliced

- 1 tablespoon of fresh ginger; peeled and sliced

- 2 tablespoons of grapeseed oil

Directions:

1. Prepare the marinade in a shallow dish or a zip-lock bag, mix vegetable stock, soy sauce, and chili powder. If you desire more spices, add ½ teaspoon of cayenne pepper. Toss the meat in the sauce and marinate for 10-15 minutes.

2. On high heat, add oil to the wok and when hot, put in ginger, broccoli, mushrooms, peas, green onions, and ¼ of the marinade, cook for about 3 minutes or until the broccoli softens. Add beef and the remaining marinade and cook until beef is browned. Serve hot.

Nutrition:

- Calories: 412
- Fat: 12 g
- Carbs: 14 g
- Protein: 24 g

Easy Pork Ribs

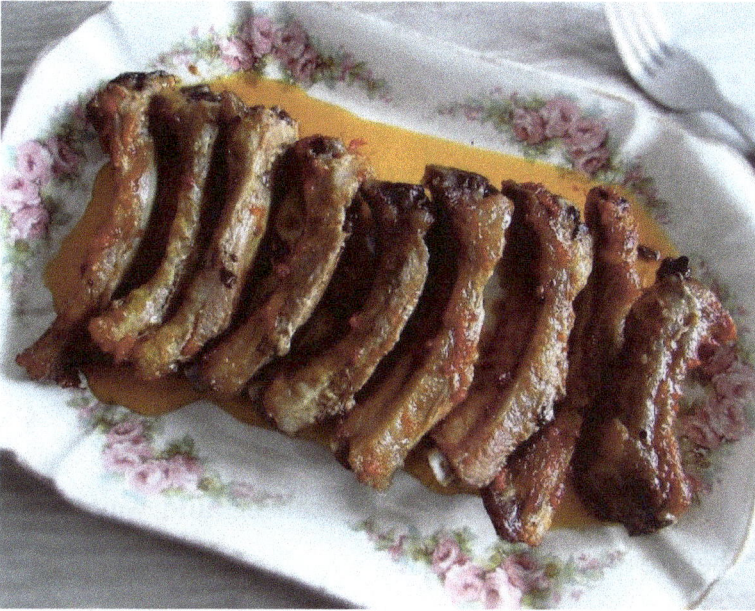

Preparation Time: 10 minutes

Cooking Time: 15 minutes

Servings: 6

Ingredients:

- 3 pounds of boneless pork ribs

- ½ cup of soy sauce

- ¼ cup of ketchup

- 2 tablespoons of olive oil
- Black pepper to taste

Directions:

1. Pour oil into your PPCXL and hit "chicken/meat," leaving the lid off.
2. When oil is hot, add ribs and roast till golden on each side.
3. In a bowl, mix black pepper, soy sauce, and ketchup.
4. Pour over ribs and seal the lid.
5. Adjust cook time to 15 minutes.
6. When the timer beeps, hit "cancel" and wait 5 minutes before quick-releasing.
7. Make sure pork is at least 145° F before serving.

Nutrition:

- Total calories: 570
- Protein: 65 g
- Carbs: 0
- Fat: 27 g
- Fiber: 0

Sesame Beef and Vegetable Stir-fry

Preparation Time: 5 minutes

Cooking Time: 30 minutes

Servings: 4

Ingredients:

- 1 pound of lean top sirloin beef; cut into strips
- 1 bunch of asparagus; bottoms cut off and stalks halved
- 1 large handful of green beans; stemmed and cut in half
- 2 onions; diced
- 1 cup of vegetable stock
- 2 tablespoons of sesame seeds
- 3 teaspoons of basil
- 2 tablespoons of grape seed oil
- 2 cups of cooked brown rice

Directions:

1. On high heat, warm grapeseed oil in wok and cook beef until it turns brown. Remove from wok.

2. Put vegetable stock in the wok and heat until it's boiling. Add asparagus, green beans, and onions and cook until soft.
3. Add beef, sesame seeds, basil, and rice and cook until everything has absorbed the vegetable stock.
4. Serve warm and enjoy!

Nutrition:

- Calories: 234
- Fat: 5 g
- Carbs: 8 g
- Protein: 44 g

Roasted Lamb with Thyme and Garlic

Preparation Time: 5 minutes

Cooking Time: 30 minutes

Servings: 4

Ingredients:

- 3 pieces of lamb
- 3 cloves of garlic
- Olive oil
- Cooking spray
- Thyme
- Salt
- Pepper

Directions:

1. Season the meat on each side.
2. Pour a little vegetable oil spray.
3. Spread crushed garlic on each bit.
4. Preheat air fryer.
5. Put the meat into fryer and add thyme.

6. Wait till meat is fully cooked.

7. Serve.

Nutrition:

- Calories: 343
- Fat: 7 g
- Carbs: 6 g
- Protein: 34 g

Garlic-Cumin and Orange Juice Marinated Steak

Preparation Time: 6 Minutes

Cooking Time: 60 Minutes

Servings: 4

Ingredients:

- ¼ cup of orange juice

- 1 teaspoon of ground cumin

- 2 pounds of skirt steak; trimmed from excess fat

- 2 tablespoons of lime juice

- 2 tablespoons of olive oil

- 4 cloves of garlic; minced

- Salt and pepper to taste

Directions:

1. Place all the ingredients in a bowl and allow to marinate in the fridge for at least 2 hours. Preheat the Cuisinart Air Fryer Oven to 390°F.
2. Place the grill pan accessory in the air fryer.

3. Grill for 15 minutes per batch and flip the meat every 8 minutes for even grilling.
4. Meanwhile, pour the marinade on a saucepan and allow to simmer for 10 minutes or until the sauce thickens.
5. Slice the meat and pour over the sauce.

Nutrition:

- Calories: 568
- Fat: 34.7 g
- Protein: 59.1 g
- Sugar: 1 g

Apple-Garlic Pork Loin

Preparation Time: 5 minutes

Cooking Time: 25 minutes

Servings: 12

Ingredients:

- One 3-pound of boneless pork loin roast
- One 12-ounce of jar of apple jelly
- 1/3 cup of water
- 1 tablespoon of Herbes de Provence
- 2 teaspoons of minced garlic

Directions:

1. Put cut of pork in your cooker. Cut in half if necessary.
2. Mix garlic, water, and jelly.
3. Pour over pork.
4. Season with Herbes de Provence.
5. Seal the lid.
6. Hit "chicken/meat" and adjust time to 25 minutes.
7. When the time is up, hit "cancel" and wait 10 minutes before quick-releasing.

8. Pork should be served at 145° F. If not cooked through yet, hit "chicken/meat" and cook with the lid off until the temperature is reached.
9. Rest for 15 minutes before slicing.

Nutrition:

- Total calories: 236
- Protein: 26 g
- Carbs: 19 g
- Fat: 6 g
- Fiber: 0

Peach-Mustard Pork Shoulder

Preparation Time: 2 minutes

Cooking Time: 55 minutes

Servings: 8

Ingredients:

- 4 pounds of pork shoulder
- 1 cup of peach
- 1 cup of white wine
- 1/3 cup of salt
- 1 tablespoon of grainy mustard

Directions:

1. Season the pork well with salt.
2. Mix mustard and peach, and rub on the pork.
3. Pour wine into cooker and add pork.
4. Seal the lid.
5. Hit "chicken/meat" and adjust time to 55 minutes.
6. When time is up, hit "cancel" and wait 10 minutes before quick-releasing.

7. Pork should be cooked to at least 145° F.

8. Move pork to a plate and cover with foil for 15 minutes before slicing and serving.

Nutrition:

- Total calories: 583
- Protein: 44 g
- Carbs: 26 g
- Fat: 32 g
- Fiber: 0

Beef Taco Fried Egg Rolls

Preparation Time: 10 Minutes

Cooking Time: 12 Minutes

Servings: 8

Ingredients:

- 1 tsp. of cilantro

- 2 chopped garlic cloves

- 1 tbsp. of olive oil

- 1 cup of shredded Mexican cheese

- ½ packet of taco seasoning

- ½ can of cilantro lime rotel

- ½ chopped onion

- 16 egg roll wrappers

- 1-pound of lean ground beef

Directions:

1. Ensure that your Cuisinart Air Fryer Oven is preheated to 400° F.

2. Add onions and garlic to a skillet, cooking till fragrant. Then add taco seasoning, pepper, salt, and beef, cooking till beef is broken up into tiny pieces and cooked thoroughly.
3. Add rotel and stir well.
4. Pour into the Oven rack/basket. Place the Rack on the middle-shelf of the Cuisinart Air Fryer Oven. Set temperature to 400°F, and set time to 8 minutes. Cook 8 minutes, flip, and cook another 4 minutes.
5. Served sprinkled with cilantro.

Nutrition:

- Calories: 348
- Fat: 11 g
- Protein: 24 g
- Sugar: 1 g

Beef with Beans

Preparation Time: 10 Minutes

Cooking Time: 13 Minutes

Servings: 4

Ingredients:

- 12 Oz. of Lean Steak
- 1 Onion; sliced
- 1 Can of Chopped Tomatoes
- 3/4 Cup of Beef Stock
- 4 tsps. of Fresh Thyme; chopped
- 1 Can of Red Kidney Beans
- Salt and Pepper to taste
- Oven Safe Bowl

Directions:

1. Preheat the Cuisinart Air Fryer Oven to 390° F.
2. Set the temperature of the Fryer Oven to 390°F, and set time to 13 minutes, then Cook for 3 minutes. Add the meat and continue cooking for five minutes.

3. Add the tomatoes and their juice, beef broth, thyme and the beans and cook for a further 5 minutes. Season with black pepper to taste.

Nutrition:

- Calories: 178
- Fat: 14 g
- Protein: 9 g
- Fiber: 0 g

Lamb cacciatore

Preparation Time: 5 minutes

Cooking Time: 1 hour

Servings: 4

Ingredients:

- 4, 41 lb. of lamb; thighs and shoulders
- 2 tablespoons of flour
- 4 anchovies in salt
- 4 tablespoons of extra virgin olive oil
- 1 sprig of rosemary
- 4 cloves of garlic
- 1 glass of vinegar or white apple

Directions:

1. Cut lamb in regular slices with a thickness of about 2 cm.
2. Wash and dry the lamb pieces. Remove the needles from the rosemary twig, wash and dry them.
3. Peel the cloves of garlic, dig slices and put them in the jar of a food processor or a blender.

4. Mix the rosemary and chop everything. Put the mixture aside.

5. Pour the oil into a large pan, let it heat and roast the pieces of lamb over high heat. When the lamb is well browned, pepper and salts it.

6. Spread the chopped garlic and rosemary over the lamb and stir.

7. Cook covered for 30-45 minutes in the Air fryer, depending on the type of lamb and the thickness of the pieces, stirring occasionally and basting with a touch predicament if the sauce too dry.

8. Desiccate and desalted the anchovies and add the fillets to lamb at the top of cooking, stir and cook a couple of minutes to dissolve.

Nutrition:

- Calories: 209
- Fat: 4.3 g
- Carbs: 20 g
- Protein: 31 g

Beef Stroganoff

Preparation Time: 10 Minutes

Cooking Time: 14 Minutes

Servings: 4

Ingredients:

- 9 Oz. of soft Beef
- 1 Onion; chopped
- 1 tbsp. of Paprika
- 3/4 Cup of Sour Cream
- Salt and Pepper to taste
- Baking Dish

Directions:

1. Preheat the Cuisinart Air Fryer Oven to 390° F.
2. Chop the meat and marinate it using paprika.
3. Add the chopped onions into the baking dish and heat for about 2 minutes in the Cuisinart Air Fryer Oven.
4. Add the meat into the dish when the onions are transparent, and cook for 5 minutes.

5. Once the meat is beginning to soften, pour in the soured cream and cook for an additional 7 minutes.
6. At this point, the liquid should have reduced. Season with salt and pepper and serve.

Nutrition:

- Calories: 254
- Fat: 21 g
- Protein: 33 g
- Fiber: 0 g

Lamb meat

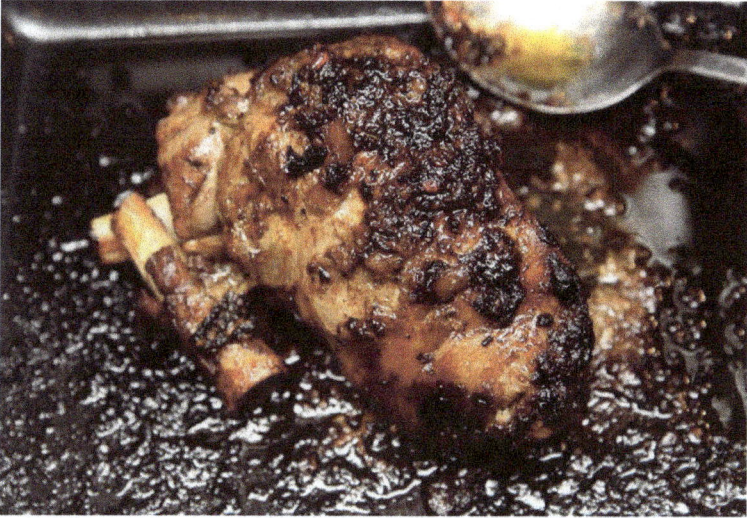

Preparation Time: 5 minutes

Cooking Time: 30 minutes

Servings: 4

Ingredients:

- Mutton any lamb

- 3 tablespoons of oil

- Curcuma; according to desire

- Saffron; as desired

- Black pepper; as desired

- Salt; according to desire

- Cup water

Directions:

1. Preheat Air fryer to 392°F;
2. Cut the meat into small pieces.
3. Sprinkle the water over the meat and add turmeric, saffron, salt, and black pepper.
4. Leave the mixture into the fryer. Wait until the meat is fully cooked and red.
5. Serve with decorations (if needed).

Nutrition:

- Calories: 203
- Fat: 9 g
- Carbs: 25 g
- Protein: 43 g

Lamb Fondue

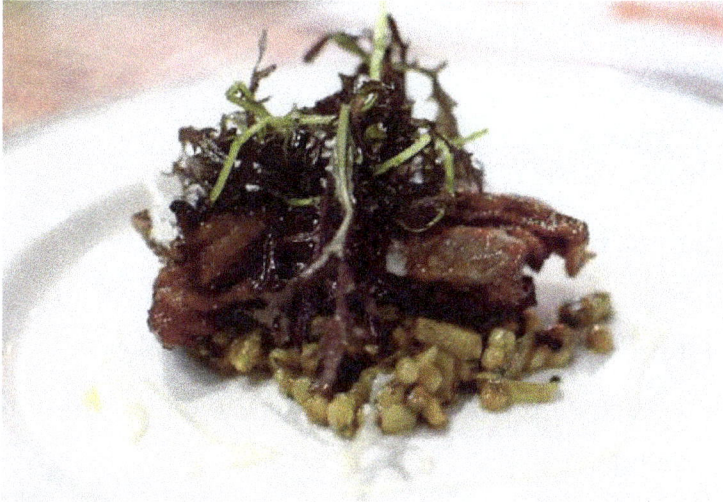

Preparation Time: 5

Cooking Time: 30

Servings: 4

Ingredients:

- 1, 32 lb. of lamb fondue pieces

- 1 eggplant

- 1 zucchini

- 1 red pepper

- 1 liter of cooking oil skewers with a diced lamb and eggplant diced zucchini
- A square of red pepper

Directions:

1. Cut the vegetables into cubes of the same size as the fondue pieces.
2. Fit mini-skewers by changing the vegetables.
3. Cooking is done at the center of the table, with a fondue machine.

Nutrition:

- Calories: 140
- Fat: 0.3 g
- Carbs: 35 g
- Protein: 3 g

Laurel Lamb with Oregano

Preparation Time: 5 minutes

Cooking Time: 30 minutes

Servings: 4

Ingredients:

- 1, 65 lb. of lamb chops
- 3 cloves garlic
- 3 leaves laurel
- A sprig of oregano
- 2 tablespoons of chopped parsley
- 1 tablespoon of fresh or dried rosemary
- C / N virgin olive oil

Directions:

1. Put the chops on a platter and sprinkle with herbs and garlic, peeled and chopped. Add salt and pepper and marinate overnight.

2. The next day put the meat in a bowl and sprinkle with olive aciete. Leave to marinate at least 4 hours. Place beat a baking dish and shut either with transparent foil.
3. Preheat air fryer to 282°F for 1 minutes
4. Lower the temperature to 338°F and set to about 15 minutes.
5. Now remove meat from the Air fryer and raise the temperature of Air fryer to 428°F.
6. Remove the wrapping and return to the Air fryer for a couple of minutes or until the meat has a golden color.
7. Serve with roasted or fried potatoes.

Nutrition:

- Calories: 206
- Fat: 21.3 g
- Carbs: 15 g
- Protein: 13 g

Airfried lamb with potatoes

Preparation Time: 5 minutes

Cooking Time: 2 hours and 30 minutes

Servings: 4

Ingredients:

- Rack of lamb
- Potatoes
- White wine
- Vegetables soup
- Garlic teeth
- Branches rosemary
- Grain Pepper
- Coarse salt

Directions:

1. Preheat the Air fryer to 392°F.
2. Place the rib in a suitable baking dish, sprinkle with coarse salt and peppercorns, then add whole garlic teeth and branches of rosemary, add oil and a few wine.

3. Put in the Air fryer and lower the temperature to 347°F.

4. Prepare a vegetable stock which can be added when it dries.

5. At that temperature, cook the rib for 2 hours. After the first hour, close up and add the potatoes, then you are ready to start serving.

Nutrition:

- Calories: 231
- Fat: 11 g
- Carbs: 12 g
- Protein: 25 g

Braised & Baked Lamb Stew

Preparation Time: 5 minutes

Cooking Time: 30 minutes

Servings: 4

Ingredients:

- 1 unit of lamb shoulder (1, 54 lb.)
- 1 piece of green pepper
- 1 clove of onion
- 1 clove of tomato
- 4 garlic cloves
- 0, 77 lb. of potato
- 1 pinch of pepper and salt
- 1 bay leaf
- ½ teaspoon of oregano
- 1 cup of white wine
- ½ cup of broth
- Meat

Directions:

1. Prepare all the ingredients. Cut lamb shoulder into two parts. Cover potatoes slightly. In a special baking pan, place in layers the pepper, tomato, onion and garlic.
2. Season with all the seasonings, wine and broth.
3. Place the lamb pieces on all the vegetables and bring to a preheated Air fryer at 356°F for 90 minutes.
4. During the frying process, check the lamb every 20-30 minutes, and turn it.
5. 15 minutes to end of cooking, open the Air fryer and place the potatoes in the pan.
6. When you finish cooking, potatoes should be softer.

Nutrition:

- Calories: 1123
- Fat: 5 g
- Carbs: 20 g
- Protein: 31 g

Lamb Meatballs with Feta

Preparation Time: 5 minutes

Cooking Time: 30 minutes

Servings: 4

Ingredients:

- 0, 33 lb. of lamb minces
- 1 slice of stale white bread; turned into fine crumbs
- 0, 11 lb. of Greek feta; crumbled
- 1 tablespoon of fresh oregano; finely chopped
- ½ tablespoon of grated lemon peel
- Freshly ground black pepper

Directions:

1. Preheat the Air Fryer to 392°F.
2. Mix the mince in a bowl with the bread crumbs, feta, oregano, lemon rind, and black pepper, thoroughly kneading everything together.
3. Cut the mixture in 10 equal portions to form round balls.

4. Place this dish in the basket inside the oven dish. Slide the basket into the Air Fryer. Set the timer to 8 minutes and bake the mince balls until they are nicely brown and done.

5. Serve the meatballs hot in a platter with tapas forks.

Nutrition:

- Calories: 300
- Fat: 2.5 g
- Carbs: 5 g
- Protein: 13 g

Garlic Lamb with Rosemary

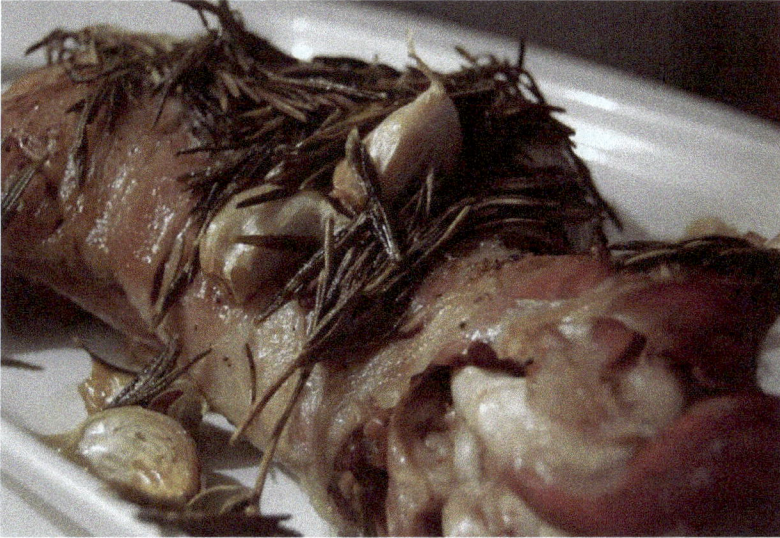

Preparation Time: 5 minutes

Cooking Time: 45 minutes

Servings: 4

Ingredients:

- 1 leg of lamb
- Branches of fresh rosemary
- Several garlic cloves
- 5 pepper (or otherwise black pepper)

- Fleur de sel

- 2 onions

- 2, 2 lb. of potatoes

- Extra virgin olive oil

Directions:

1. Preheat the Air fryer to 356°F.
2. Remove the blade bone of the lamb. Remove excess fat.
3. Dry the piece of blood residues. If you removed the bone, add salt, and pepper inside, then close and tie round with kitchen string. Peel the garlic cloves and cut 3 pieces lengthwise. Wash the rosemary.
4. Add garlic and rosemary all over the outer surface of the lamb leg. To do this, make a deep incision with a knife and put inside a bit of garlic and a sprig of rosemary. Coat the surface generously with sea salt and 5 peppers.
5. Peel the potatoes, rinse, and cut thick slices of 5 mm thickness. Peel onions and cut them into thick equal slices.
6. Grease the bottom of the baking tray with olive oil. Place the potato slices on the tray and spread the onion on top.
7. Place the lamb with garlic and rosemary in the center and sprinkle with olive oil.

8. Bake each 1 lb. of meat at medium heat for 15 minutes so that it is a little done and 20 to 25 minutes per 1, 1 lb to the point that it is either done.
9. A half cooking, add half glass of water to the potato or a little more, as needed.
10. If the surface is browning too quickly, cover with baking paper. Optionally, 15 minutes before the end of cooking, sprinkle top with melted butter and finish uncovered.

Nutrition:

- Calories: 365
- Fat: 21 g
- Carbs: 11 g
- Protein: 15 g

Roasted Lamb with Honey

Preparation Time: 5 minutes

Cooking Time: 30 minutes

Servings: 4

Ingredients:

- 1, 32 lb. of lamb
- 2 tablespoons of mustard tarragon
- 2 tablespoons of rosemary honey
- 2 tablespoons of soy
- 1 teaspoon of rosemary; chopped
- 2 cloves of garlic; minced
- C / N Extra virgin olive
- 0, 88 lb of potatoes; peeled and chopped
- Salt and black pepper

Directions:

1. Put the meat to macerate the night before with mustard, honey, soy, chopped rosemary, garlic, 1 chorretón oil, salt and pepper.

2. Cook the potatoes and put aside.

3. Place meat in a preheated Air fryer at 392°F for 20 minutes. Remove and add the potatoes.

4. Return meat to Air fryer and lower the temperature to 338°F. When the meat is cooked, remove and serve with potatoes.

Nutrition:

- Calories: 243
- Fat: 22 g
- Carbs: 13 g
- Protein: 20 g

Baked Patties

Preparation Time: 10 minutes

Cooking Time: 15 minutes

Servings: 4

Ingredients:

- 1 lb. of ground lamb
- 1 teaspoon of ground coriander
- 1 teaspoon of ground cumin
- ¼ cup of fresh parsley; chopped
- ¼ cup of onion; minced
- ¼ teaspoon of cayenne pepper
- ½ teaspoon of ground allspice
- 1 teaspoon of ground cinnamon
- 1 tablespoon of garlic; minced
- ¼ teaspoon of pepper
- 1 teaspoon of kosher salt

Directions:

1. Preheat the oven to 450° F.
2. Add all the ingredients into a big bowl and blend until well mixed.
3. Make small meatballs from meat mixture and place on a baking tray and lightly flatten the meatballs with the back of a spoon.
4. Bake in preheated oven for 12-15 minutes.
5. Serve and enjoy.

Nutrition:

- Calories: 112
- Fat: 4.3 g
- Carbohydrates: 1.3 g
- Sugar: 0.2 g
- Protein: 16 g
- Cholesterol: 51 mg

Lamb tagine

Servings: 4

Ingredients:

- 1.32 lb. of lamb shoulder
- oz. of white wine
- 0.088 lb. of pitted black olives
- 04 ml of water
- 0.033 lb. of fresh ginger
- 0.015 lb. of lemon zest
- 1 spoon of garlic powder
- 1 spoon of oil
- 1 spoon of parsley
- 1 spoon of coriander
- 1 dose of saffron
- 1 spoon of maizena
- Salt
- Pepper

Directions:

1. Slice the lamb into cubes of 3-4 cm and coat the pieces of Maizena. Chop the ginger.
2. In a bowl, mix the wine and water.
3. Grate the lemon
4. Put the olives, ginger, lemon peel, parsley, coriander, saffron, and garlic in air fryer—handle side of tank.
5. Arrange the lamb in the bowl opposite the handle. Pour the mixture over the spices. Spread the oil over the lamb. Close the hood.
6. Start cooking.

Nutrition:

- Calories: 105
- Fat: 29 g
- Carbs: 2 g
- Protein: 23 g

Lamb chops

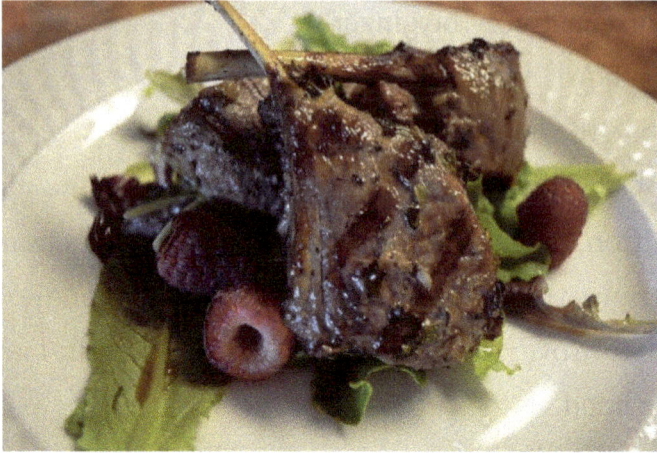

Preparation Time: 10 minutes

Cooking Time: 25 minutes

Servings: 4

Ingredients:

- Oregano
- Thyme
- Garlic
- Salt
- Pepper

Directions:

1. Cut the vegetables into cubes of the same size of fondue pieces.
2. Fit mini-skewers by changing the vegetables.
3. Cooking is completed at the middle of the table, with a fondue machine.

Nutrition:

- Calories: 279
- Fat: 11 g
- Carbs: 13 g
- Protein: 43 g

Breaded and crispy lamb chops

Preparation Time: 5 minutes

Cooking Time: 30 minutes

Servings: 4

Ingredients:

- 2 eggs
- 8 lean lamb chops
- 0.044 lb. of flour
- 0.44 lb. of breadcrumbs (made of crumbled breadcrumbs)
- 52.79 oz. of cooking oil

Directions:

1. Beat the eggs with salt and pepper.
2. Pass the lamb chops, first in the flour, and then in the eggs, and eventually in the bread crumbs. To get a thicker crust, pass the chops again in the eggs and then in the bread crumbs.
3. Heat the oil in the air fryer at approx. 338°F.

4. Fry the chops until they're golden brown.

5. Allow them drain on paper towels, sprinkle with salt and pepper to taste and store (uncovered) in an oven.

Nutrition:

- Calories: 142
- Fat: 9.3 g
- Carbs: 5 g
- Protein: 53 g

Beef Patties

Preparation Time: 10 minutes

Cooking Time: 8 minutes

Servings: 5

Ingredients:

- 1 lb. of ground beef
- 1 egg; lightly beaten
- 3 tablespoon of almond flour
- 1 small onion; grated
- 2 tablespoon of fresh parsley; chopped
- 1 teaspoon of dry oregano
- 1 teaspoon of dry mint
- Pepper
- Salt

Directions:

1. Using a sharp knife, make small cuts all over the meat then insert garlic slivers into the cuts.

2. In a small bowl, mix together marjoram, thyme, oregano, pepper, salt, and rub all over the roast lamb.
3. Place roast lamb into the slow cooker.
4. Cover and cook on low for 8 hours.
5. Serve and enjoy.

Nutrition:

- Calories: 188
- Fat: 6.6 g
- Carbohydrates: 1.7 g
- Sugar: 0.7 g
- Protein: 28.9 g
- Cholesterol: 114 mg

Tender & Juicy Lamb Roast

Preparation Time: 10 minutes

Cooking Time: 8 hours

Servings: 8

Ingredients:

- 4 lbs. of lamb roast; boneless

- ½ teaspoon of thyme

- 1 teaspoon of oregano

- 4 garlic cloves; cut into slivers
- ½ teaspoon of marjoram
- ¼ teaspoon of pepper
- 2 teaspoons of salt

Directions:

1. Using a sharp knife, make small cuts all over meat then insert garlic slivers into the cuts.
2. In a small bowl, mix together the marjoram, thyme, oregano, pepper, salt, and rub all over lamb roast.
3. Place lamb roast into the slow cooker.
4. Cover and cook on low for 8 hours.
5. Serve and enjoy.

Nutrition:

- Calories: 605
- Fat: 48 g
- Carbohydrates: 0.7 g
- Sugar: 1 g
- Protein: 36 g
- Cholesterol: 160 mg

Basil Cheese Pork Roast

Preparation Time: 10 minutes

Cooking Time: 6 hours

Servings: 8

Ingredients:

- 2 lbs. of lean pork roast, boneless
- 1 teaspoon of garlic powder
- 1 tablespoon of parsley
- ½ cup of cheddar cheese; grated
- 30 oz. of can tomatoes; diced
- 1 teaspoon of dried oregano
- 1 teaspoon of dried basil
- Pepper
- Salt

Directions:

1. Add the meat into the crock pot.
2. Mix together tomatoes, oregano, basil, garlic powder, parsley, cheese, pepper, salt, and pour over the meat.

3. Cover and cook on low for 6 hours.
4. Serve and enjoy.

Nutrition:

- Calories: 260
- Fat: 9 g
- Carbohydrates: 5.5 g
- Sugar: 3.5 g
- Protein: 35 g
- Cholesterol: 97 mg

Feta Lamb Patties

Preparation Time: 10 minutes

Cooking Time: 12 minutes

Servings: 4

Ingredients:

- 1 lb. of ground lamb
- 1/2 teaspoon of garlic powder
- 1/2 cup of feta cheese; crumbled
- 1/4 cup of mint leaves; chopped
- 1/4 cup of roasted red pepper; chopped
- 1/4 cup of onion; chopped
- Pepper
- Salt

Directions:

1. Add all ingredients into a bowl and blend until well mixed.
2. Spray pan with cooking spray and heat over medium-high heat.

3. Make small patties from meat mixture and place on hot pan and cook for 6-7 minutes on all sides.

4. Serve and enjoy.

Nutrition:

- Calories: 270
- Fat: 12 g
- Carbohydrates: 2.9 g
- Sugar: 1.7 g
- Protein: 34.9 g
- Cholesterol: 119 mg

Cheesy Ground Beef and Mac Taco Casserole

Preparation Time: 10 Minutes

Cooking Time: 25 Minutes

Servings: 5

Ingredients:

- 1-ounce of shredded Cheddar cheese
- 1-ounce of shredded Monterey Jack cheese
- 2 tablespoons of chopped green onions
- 1/2 (10.75 ounce) can of condensed tomato soup
- 1/2-pound of lean ground beef
- 1/2 cup of crushed tortilla chips
- 1/4-pound of macaroni; cooked according to manufacturer's
- 1/4 cup of chopped onion
- 1/4 cup of sour cream (optional)
- 1/2 (1.25 ounce) package of taco seasoning mix
- 1/2 (14.5 ounce) can of diced tomatoes

Directions:

1. Lightly grease baking pan of air fryer with cooking spray. Add onion and ground beef. Cook on 360°F for 10 minutes. Halfway into cooking time, stir and crumble ground beef.
2. Add taco seasoning, diced tomatoes, and tomato soup. Mix well in pasta.
3. Sprinkle crushed tortilla chips. Sprinkle cheese.
4. Cook for 15 minutes at 390°F or until tops are lightly browned and cheese is melted.
5. Serve and enjoy.

Nutrition:

- Calories: 329
- Fat: 17 g
- Protein: 15.6 g

Beefy Steak Topped with Chimichurri Sauce

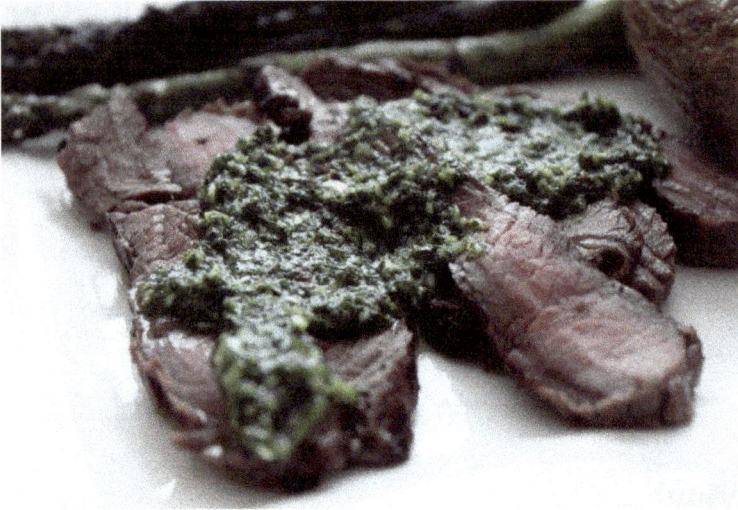

Preparation Time: 5 Minutes

Cooking Time: 60 Minutes

Servings: 6

Ingredients:

- 1 cup of commercial chimichurri

- 3 pounds of steak

- Salt and pepper to taste

Directions:

1. Place all ingredients in a Ziploc bag and marinate in the fridge for 2 hours.
2. Preheat the air fryer to 390°F.
3. Place the grill pan accessory in the air fryer.
4. Grill the skirt steak for 20 minutes per batch.
5. Flip the steak every 10 minutes for even grilling.

Nutrition:

- Calories: 507
- Fat: 27 g
- Protein: 63 g

www.ingramcontent.com/pod-product-compliance
Lightning Source LLC
Chambersburg PA
CBHW050747030426
42336CB00012B/1702